Introduction

'Let us therefore follow things which make for peace, and things wherewith one may edify another'

Romans 15:19

When Age Concern England asked me to write this book, I was delighted. We both feel that, although so many books have been published for the elderly – I have already written one myself – these are mostly for the fairly robust. There remains one group who seems to have been neglected.

They are older people who either live alone, or if they live with their family, who may be working, spend a lot of time by themselves. Also there are quite a few people living in old people's homes who are shy of joining in activities. They are the ones who, when games or discussions are going on say 'I'll just watch, thank you', or just 'No thank you', and that's the end of that. These people therefore miss much stimulation of body and mind, and gradually become more frail in health, and use their thinking capacities less and less; even their voices become hardly audible. Then they may be pushed aside, or even regarded as a nuisance.

We hope that this book may be acceptable to them – either to read alone or to share with someone else, so that they may arrest their growing weakness, and begin to enjoy a fuller life again.

People will probably dip into this book from time to time, rather than read it straight through. For this reason I repeat, from various angles and under different headings, important ideas like proper breathing, diet, walking etc. I hope this will not be annoying.

Sometimes people are happy, healthy and joining in all kinds of activities, when some dread happening lays them low; the death of a close family member, financial change or a serious illness. Though they live through it, the experience devastates them so much that they are changed and become what is known as 'the old and frail'.

But they can come alive again with gentle understanding help. That is what we hope this book will supply. They really are 'Very Important People'.

Let us appreciate their worth, for they are the people who, during their long lives, have helped to win two world wars which were fought to preserve the free way of life we all enjoy.

They have often held positions of great responsibility and given generous public service; or they may have known deprivation, both in living conditions and in their working lives. They are certainly the fathers and mothers of all succeeding generations.

Let us help them now to realise that they are still wanted, honoured, loved, and help them to rebuild their self-esteem, general health and happiness.

Foreword

In the Introduction, I tried to explain why I had written this book. Now I would like to say a few words to those of whom I have tried to write. I have been thinking of you so much for months, as I was writing, that I feel we are already friends.

Some readers may be thinking 'It's all very well for her to talk. It's probably easy for her.' I will therefore tell you I am 82 years of age, and I live alone. I have had four hip operations and years of arthritis in my spine. I have one leg now three and a half inches shorter than the other because I have no hip joint on that side, and part of the leg bone removed due to a bone infection. There is an artificial hip on the other side. I have had cancer, and following an operation for that I am well and have no pain. I have, however, rather steep front door steps – nine of them. But I find if I go down backwards, holding on to the rail, I can manage well. I walk with a crutch on one side and a stick on the other, and do exercises every day for my back and legs.

Much research is being done in many parts of the

world on Gerontology ie, the study of ageing. One conclusion is that the reason why some older people appear to have lost their thinking capacity and general activity, is due to the way they live, and often because 'they simply do not use the brain power they have'.

So don't listen to the people who tell you, you must expect to degenerate because you will lose your brain cells with increasing age. You have over twelve BILLION cells in your nervous system when you are born, so you can afford to get rid of a few all through life and have plenty left to think with *if you use them*.

So that is what I have tried to do. To encourage you to keep on using your life and experimenting, I want to remind you that we are not composed only of body and emotion, but also mind and spirit too. If our bodies are sometimes not as full of energy as they once were, or are giving us some pain or disability and perhaps causing us emotional annoyance or even distress, then our minds and spirits are still at our disposal to energise our lives.

If for any reason anyone is prevented from normal activity, their health always gets into a low state, and they are then more likely to become unhappy and ill. Our bodies maintain health by all parts working smoothly, and for this we need good food, suitable exercise and rest, and a free supply of blood to and from all parts.

This is why I have suggested several ways of movement and reminded you often of good breathing.

All this affects your brain and heart. These are the centres of your body health, and each has a system of alternating activity and rest. Your brain likes to work hard at interesting thoughts and then to have sleep to recover.

Your heart works extremely hard to pump your blood all round your body including your brain and lungs seventy-two times every minute! Yes, seventy-two times every minute!

This is such an immense performance that its resting period actually amounts to more than its active time (0.3 work and 0.5 rest per second). So that if you live for a hundred years, your heart will have rested more than fifty years!

As I believe in following quite humbly the rules of how the body naturally performs rather than dictating to it, I have put in lots of activity for mind and muscles, also rhythmn and relaxation.

I hope you will soon feel the excellent results that other people have. Your eyes will sparkle, your breathing be easier, your brain more active and you will feel you really can once again enjoy life.

Laura Mitchell
May 1988

Your Upper Half and Lower Half

▤ Hands, faces and breathing

■ Hands and faces

Have you noticed that our hands are always trying to curl up? Some people even roll tissue in their hands because someone has told them to 'keep your fingers moving'. Yes – moving – but not always inwards please, they are there already.

Instead try doing this.

Rest your elbows comfortably on a table or the arms of your chair. Now press your wrists together in front of you and then stretch your hands so that each finger rests on the opposite finger.

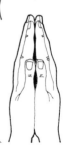

Now lift your elbows and press your fingers together so that they are touching all along. Your two thumbs face your face lying beside each other.

Do all this very gently and easily. Hands are delicate even if they can do strong work. If we don't look after them, the joints can become swollen and go out of shape.

Do you put some soft, sweet-smelling cream on your hands every day? Please do. After washing is a good time, and the sweet smell will give you pleasure and make you smile.

Did you know smiling is the best beauty treatment? It takes out all the lines on your face that run downwards, and lifts them upwards.

Hold a mirror close up in front of your face. Above your upper lip you will probably see little lines running from your nose towards your top lip. Most older people have them. I know I do. Now smile and you will see the corners of your lips lift up and the little lines disappear.

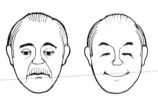

Now frown and purse your lips together and see how unpleasant you look and all the disagreeable lines reappear. Do you do that often?

Sometimes I see myself frowning if I am thinking hard. But having seen how awful I look when I do that, I always now make myself smile instead.

I just think of someone I am fond of, and smiling is quite easy. Sometimes I am told, 'you don't look your age'. I'm eighty-two. I think it must be because I have learned to smile instead of frowning. Try it.

Now let's go back to the hands again. Lay the back of your hand on your knee and bend all your fingers inwards to touch the palm just where it joins your fingers. Get them as close as possible then press and release them against your palm in little gentle bouncing movements. Don't press them in with your other hand and never, never allow anyone else to force your joints. This can damage them. If you use your own muscles they will protect your joints.

Now open your hands out wide so the fingers and thumbs are straight and you make as wide a space as you can between each of them. Go on, really work at it! And then bring your finger tips in again to touch the same place on your palm. Repeat all that if you wish. Have a rest.

When you are ready, bend your fingers once again. This time try to touch the cushion of flesh in your palm just above your wrist where your thumb begins. Again, try little pressing movements with the pads of your fingers, while your nails are showing above.

Open out again. Then repeat all that if you wish. Then hang your arm over the side of your chair, and shake your hand as though you were trying to make it fall off your wrist. Have a rest.

Lastly, make a fist with your thumb inside your fingers, then stretch fingers and thumb out wide, then make a fist with your thumb outside your fingers. Repeat each quickly six times in turn. This makes you think very fast and that is good for everyone. When you wish, do all that with your other hand.

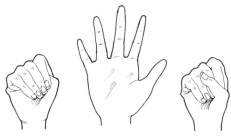

Here is a game to play with your fingers which you can do by yourself. You need some safety pins, some ordinary pins and a pin cushion. It is a good idea to have the pins on a plate, otherwise they scatter all over the place.

Pick up a pin and push it into the pin cushion till only the head shows. You are going to make the first initial of your name by the pins. For instance, if your first name was Isabel, you would make a picture like this then if you wish you can decorate it with safety pins.

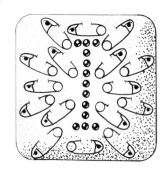

They must all be closed while lying on the plate.

You select one, whichever size you want, carefully open it and slide it into the pin cushion, so that you can close it up again. Be careful not to prick yourself. You could make a circle of safety pins around your initial, or any other pattern you fancy. Handling pins requires very exact control by your fingers, so you are really caring for your joints, skin, muscles and all the nerves from your brain to your fingers and from your fingers to your brain, as you do the job.

I wonder if you have heard the expression *'USE IT, OR LOSE IT'* ? It is quite true, I'm sure you don't want to become one of those people who sit idle all day with useless hands lying still, and probably aching, in their laps. Use them!

Do you wash something every day? A pair of socks or stockings, a pair of pants or a handkerchief? This is the most comfortable way to keep your hands alive and active. Try to wring out some things. Wringing in both directions is good for elbows. You will be pleased with yourself as you hang your little washing up to dry. You will have given help to all your arm joints as well as your self respect. Nothing like doing a little job for yourself or someone else, to make you feel really happy and satisfied!

A word about your shoulders. Do you ever wonder why you have arms and shoulder joints? Well, it is so that you can move you hands about! So shoulders and hands go together. If you have weakness in one, you will tend to have a weakness in the other. If one aches, soon the other will begin to ache. Here is how to get rid of both the weakness and the aches. Raise your arm above your head. Hold it there and push you hand up towards the ceiling several times. Then drop your hand quickly to smack your thigh, then throw it up again above your head.

Try and repeat this a few times. You will find it gets easier as you do it. When you feel you can, try doing it with both hands, and make them clap above your head and then slap both your thighs when you bring them down. Then make your head follow your hands' direction upwards and downwards. Look at your hands. Go on, make as much noise as you can, and you might like to sing a song you like as you do it, so you get a good rhythm going.

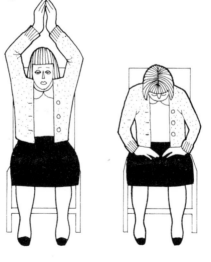

UP, DOWN, UP, DOWN, UP, DOWN. You will soon find you are out of breath but don't worry, that is very good for you. When you hurry up your breathing, your heart gets stronger and your blood is hurried round your body. Then you get more oxygen to your brain and this makes you feel better and able to think more clearly. This is always a good idea. Let us look at breathing a little more. (For more on breathing see pages 33,39,41).

■ Breathing

When you breathe in you fill your lungs with fresh air. At least I hope it is fresh, and not stale old air in a room where the windows are never opened. This is one reason why you should go out every day, even if only to stand on a balcony or the front steps or the patio at the back door. Your lungs are made of very tiny little blood vessels as fine as a hair, lying in spaces for the air to fill up. If you spread out all these blood vessels flat, there are so many of them they would cover a tennis court. Think of that! A whole tennis court filled with fresh air is inside your chest when you breathe in deeply!

Breathe in through your nose, because lining it there are very small hairs to trap any dust in the air and also an arrangement of warm blood vessels to heat the air as it passes along just like central heating. This is why you should not breathe through your mouth because it doesn't have all this. Mouths are for eating, talking and laughing; noses are for breathing and smelling.

When you breathe in, make your tummy swell out and your chest get bigger. I hope you can feel your ribs on either side open out towards your armpits just like a bird's wings open when it flies.

Now breathe out through your nose and feel how your ribs fall in again and your tummy gets smaller. You can pull your tummy tighter if you like, we all want small tummies, don't we?

Let your breathing settle and then try again. This time, put your hands on your ribs so your little fingers are on your waist at either side. As you balloon out your tummy and chest when you breathe in, you will feel your hands lifted forwards and sideways. When you breathe out, give a little squeeze with your hands on your chest as you pull in your tummy. You can repeat another deep breath but no more. Twice is enough at a time.

It is often a good idea to get up before every meal. Go to the lavatory, empty your bladder, wash your hands and do two deep breaths; if possible in the open air, but certainly in an open space like the hall or corridor.

When you sit down to eat, you will find you have a better appetite for your meal and a clearer brain to chat to your neighbour as you eat. Or if you are alone, turn on the radio and listen to that as you eat; I am often alone for my meals and then I always do that. And I find I'm talking to the people on the wireless as though I know them. Meals are times for chatting. It is very dull just to sit there eating in complete silence.

▤ Sitting, standing and walking

Do you know that most falls that people have in their homes take place after they have been sitting still for some time? A fall is what most old people dread, so let us see what we can do to prevent us having that horrid experience with perhaps a broken arm or leg into the bargain.

■ Sitting

Try never to sit for more than half an hour at a time. It is prolonged idleness that makes all our muscles weak and floppy, and then unable to control our weight when eventually we do try to stand up.

Don't allow yourself to be padded in with too many cushions, especially if you are sitting in one of those low armchairs, so that you disappear into it and practically need a crane to get out of it.

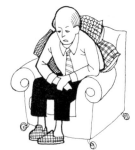

everything WRONG

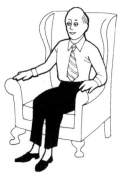

everything RIGHT

You should be able to wriggle about in your chair, lean forward to talk to other people and able to turn round to see out of the window, and to do the 'Holding and shouting' (page 27) when you feel like it.

When you decide to stand up, pay some attention to what you are doing. Wriggle to the front of the chair, grasping the arms of the chair to help you.

Both feet should be flat on the floor, comfortably apart and your head should be held high with your nose facing forward. When you do this your back muscles will be getting ready to lift you upright.

Now make several little trial lifts upward.

All at the same time	Press feet down	*UP YOU GO*
	Press hands on chair arms	*AND SINK*
	Lift head	*AGAIN*

When you have done this several times, each lift rising a few inches, you are ready for the final rise. Press hands and feet as before and *with your head up* rise by clenching your buttocks strongly and you will find you are standing: you will feel very proud and in control of yourself when you do this, very different from being hauled about like a parcel by other people.

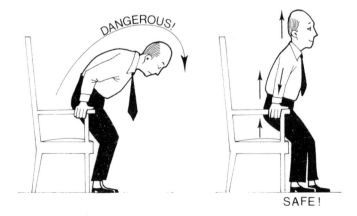

DANGEROUS!

SAFE!

Now you can take your stick(s) and walk away, or stay standing if you wish.

■ Standing

You would think that once you have got up from your chair, you were in a safe standing position. Yes, but few people stand in such a way that the whole body is comfortable and able to function well.

The diagram shows what should happen, so please study it well. It is not difficult to do, and as you gain control of yourself, you feel that splendid sensation of health and safety.

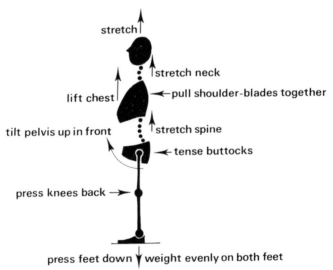

By stretching your whole spine you free all the nerves so that they work more easily. By lifting your chest, you breathe freely and you take the pressure off your abdomen and its contents so your digestion improves.

When you pull your shoulder blades together, tense your buttocks, press your knees back and place your feet firmly onto the floor, you really have control of your weight.

Be sure you put your weight evenly on both feet whether you use a stick or not. Some people put all their weight on one leg, or even on their stick so that they gradually get weaker and become in danger of falling.

Be aware of resting your weight against furniture, for example, the kitchen table when cooking, or the hand basin if washing. Stand secure, swaying gently and safely balanced on your two feet.

■ Walking

Of course you are wearing proper shoes and not soft bedroom slippers. This allows you to walk heel toe, heel toe, instead of shuffling forward with your feet flat on the floor and no movement in your ankles at all. Lift your knee as you bring the back leg forward to put your heel down and, if you use a stick, it should be coming forward at the same time on the opposite side.

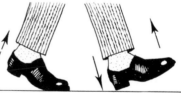

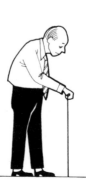

WRONG

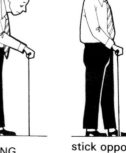

stick opposite
forward leg

If you use two sticks they move one at a time with the opposite leg. This is to preserve your human two-legged walk. Otherwise you move like a horse with four legs, one after the other. You should only allow yourself to do this if you are really very 'old and frail', because although it is safe, it is weakening because you don't use your legs and back properly and your sense of balance stops working.

If you are walking with the support of some other person, see they are alongside you, not in front. You take their arm, or rest your hand on their shoulder, rather than let them grasp you, which some people are apt to do, and upset your balance. How often I have nearly been knocked over by some willing but inexperienced person suddenly enveloping me because they see I use a stick!

You must remain in charge of your walking. Do not allow someone else to hurry you along, or else to dawdle unnecessarily.

▤ Patting and stroking

(sitting in an upright chair)

Let us try *patting and stroking*. You lift your right hand. You bend the fingers and thumb just enough to make it into a little bowl and then you pat your other shoulder with this, flapping it up and down at your wrist. Now pat all down your arm. It should be a comfortable, pleasant feeling. Pat down your arm

from your shoulder to your hand and up again.
When you feel it nice and warm, change to
stroking it. Like this:

Stretch out your fingers and thumb and beginning
at your other shoulder once more, curve your hand
cosily around your shoulder and then continue
stroking right down your arm over your hand.
Then stroke all the way up
again on the other side of
your arm. That means if you
began at your shoulder you
would stroke all the way
down on the outside and then
all the way up on the inside.
Always finish curving your
hand all around your shoulder
in a comforting circle.
Shoulders often ache and this
stroking is very soothing, and
the patting brings blood to
your whole arm to heat it up.

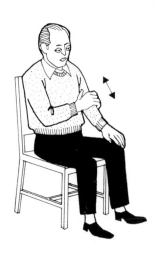

Next, repeat with your left hand, helping your
other arm to feel better. You can sing if you like
when you are doing this. I think you'll enjoy it
even more if you are singing one of your favourite
songs and keeping time.

Now you go on to patting your legs. In the same
way as before, cup your right hand and bend across
to pat your other leg, and go on patting as far
down as you can manage. Pat upwards again, and
then go on patting up and down seeing if you can
reach further down each time. When you wish,

you can change to stroking
down the outside of your leg
and up the inside, just as you
stroked your arm.

Then you can turn the other
way and using your left hand,
treat your opposite leg in
exactly the same way.

By now I hope you will be
glowing all over with your legs and
arms feeling warm and soothed. Maybe you feel a
bit breathless and that is a good thing. Doctors tell
us that we all ought to work our bodies every day
enough to be a bit breathless. This makes our
lungs work better, getting rid of stale air and
filling them full of fresh air. Just sit calmly,
letting your breath come back to normal in its
own time, and then take a couple of easy big
breaths, letting your tummy expand as you
breathe through your nose, then your ribs move
out like the wings on a bird on either side of you
as you continue to breathe in. When you are
ready, breathe out again through your nose and
you will feel your ribs fall down again and your
tummy flatten. It is a good idea to pull your
tummy inwards when this happens. I think all of
us wish we had a flatter tummy as we had when
we were young. This movement of our tummies
forwards and then inwards helps to prevent
constipation also.

Here is a fun 'pat and stroke' to do, which you
may already know.

You pat the top of your head with one hand and at the same time stroke your tummy round in a circle with the other hand.

The trick is to begin patting your head, and when you have the rhythm going, join in the same rhythm with your other hand on your tummy. You might try doing it with a friend opposite each other and have a good laugh.

Then you can go on to 'mirror-following'. One of you makes any kind of hand and arm movements, and the opposite person pretends he or she is a mirror and does exactly the same movement at the same time. It is quite fascinating to do. Then you swop who leads and who follows and you can use music from the radio if you like. You'll be surprised how versatile you can be and how graceful!

▤ Catching a moth for strong arms

Think how often we have all seen a moth fluttering about and how we have rushed to catch it before it got in among our woollies with the resulting holes that ruin our clothes.

Now imagine you see a moth and stretch out your hands to catch it in the air. Clap your hands hard

together as you imagine
it moving all round you,
above, to the side, below,
up again. The moth
always seems just to
manage to get away.
Imagine it fluttering all
around and you are now
getting desperate to catch it.
Stretch up high, lean over sideways and
downwards and each time say *'BANG'* as loud as
you can when you bang your hands together,
trying to hit that fluttering moth. Have a rest and
try again later.

Holding and shouting

Today I am going to suggest some amazingly easy
ways of getting your legs stronger for standing and
walking; also your arms for washing and dressing
plus voice training. No, not training as people do
for singing opera, I wouldn't know how to do that.

But I have noticed that often older people who do
not talk very much, begin to lose their voices and
tend to speak in a whisper. Also their breathing
begins to get very shallow and that may lead to
chest complaints.

So what we are going to do will make you able to
walk and talk better, so that you can go out and
about and enjoy yourself more.

Sit on a fairly upright chair if possible, or just try where you are now. Raise one leg, straightening it at the knee with your foot towards the ceiling.

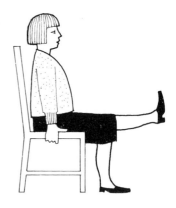

That is all you do. You just keep it up there, very stiff and very still. If you have a minute hand on your watch, time how many seconds you can hold it there.

When I began to do this, I could only hold my leg up for thirty seconds. Now, after doing it for six months most days, I can hold it easily for two minutes, and my legs are much stronger for walking and gardening. I garden a lot, (keep your leg up), and as I cannot kneel because my right thigh is three inches shorter than my left, I have to weed and plant standing, or sitting and bending forwards. Yesterday I spent two hours planting and weeding.

You need strong legs to be safe standing and bending forwards to pick up anything from the floor, without falling over. If you want to pick up a milk bottle or anything you have dropped without falling over, you must give your muscles extra work to do, to keep yourself safe. Have you still got your leg quite straight in front of you? Or have you put it down? That's all right, just do what you can.

Now straighten out your other leg and call out loudly as you can *'I AM MRS SMITH'* or *'I AM MRS BROWN'*, or whatever name you like to be called by, and count on your fingers the number of times you can call out before you have to lower your foot. You should really shout.

All this is quite difficult to do at the same time, so you are really working very hard both in your brain and body. Therefore only do it as long as you wish and then stop. You can do the leg holding at any odd time, even if it is not convenient to do the shouting. Try doing it watching television, waiting for a meal, sitting reading or sewing. You will find opportunities for yourself.

Now the arms. You raise your arm to the level of your shoulders then pull it backwards a little and just hold it there. Do your shouting and this time choose your own words. Shout anything you like and count on your other hand, tapping your knee with your fingers so that you

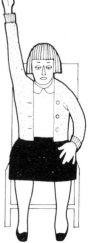

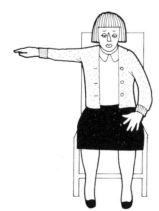

know how long you have been able to hold your arm up, before you had to drop it – five taps or ten or fifteen taps. Then you do all that again with your other arm.

Later, if you like, you can change the position of your arm to be above your head. You may find this a little easier. You have to do both positions to strengthen your whole arm.

Here is another way to make your legs really strong enough to carry you about.

Stand up and hold on to some strong piece of furniture with both hands. Now 'mark time' as quickly as you can – really fast – *RIGHT, LEFT, RIGHT, LEFT, LIFTING YOUR KNEES*.

Then put your feet together, straighten your knees and rise onto your toes (hold on tight), lower your bottom by bending your knees turned outwards, only as much as seems safe, and then straighten your knees up again and raise your heels. Lower your heels.

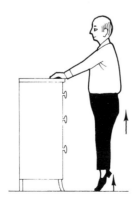 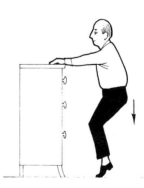

You may remember this from your school days as 'heel raising, knee bending'. Do it about two or three times, gradually increasing the number of times as you get stronger. I can now do it ten times (said she showing off!). You show off too, and write and tell me when you reach ten times and you can hold your knee stiff and your arm up for two full minutes.

Your Middle

 ## Rocking and breathing
(sitting down)

Rock your body forwards and then backwards to touch the back of the chair. As you do so say 'forwards and backwards', repeated in time to the rocking. You will find this very soothing. Then rock your body sideways as far as you comfortably can; as you do so repeat the words *'OVER AND OVER AGAIN'* as you rock from side to side.

Stop whenever you want.

Now you are going to rock each leg. You keep your toes on the ground and bend your foot so your heel lifts up and your knee rises into the air. Do this with alternate legs, one after the other, and say *'UP AND UP AND UP AND UP'*, keeping time as you raise each heel and knee.

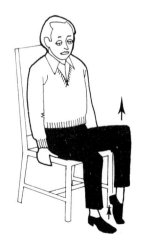

The last parts of you to rock are your arms. You clasp your arms together loosely in front of your chest, then you rock them from side to side, pushing them as far as you can to each side saying as loudly as you can as you do so, 'ROCK, ROCK, ROCK, ROCK'.

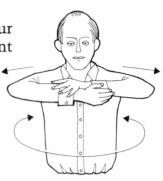

You can turn your whole body if you like as you rock your arms. It is like dancing, so if you prefer to sing a song from your dancing days, do just that as loudly as you can. Stop.

Now I hope you are feeling a bit breathless, so let's do the deep breathing that by now you know so well, I hope.

Because we all have to breathe all the time to stay alive, it is a good idea to take a few deep breaths from time to time so that your lungs get really fully stretched, and so more air goes into them and you get rid of more and more stale air, full of rubbish from your blood.

Remember how much your brain needs oxygen to keep working well, so here goes.

Put your spread out hands gently on the sides of your chest and breathe in by ballooning forward your tummy and opening out your ribs under your hands. Do it easily and gently and when you feel you have done enough, breathe out and press your hands against your ribs. Do it once more only.

▤ Eating and drinking

I hope you 'enjoy your food'. Eating and drinking are part of the pleasures of life, and so are very, very important for us all.

If you live alone, I hope you have a pretty table to sit at and that you use your best china and glass and any silver you have.

I do this, and although I usually eat at my kitchen table when I am alone, it is carefully set and with often a small vase of flowers I bring in from the garden, summer or winter.

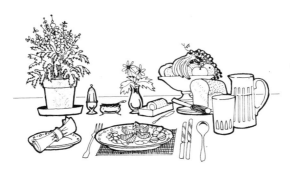

There is always a scented geranium in a pot. It has a bitter sweet smell which I always enjoy, and when I am eating a salad I may put in a leaf to mix with the lemon and olive oil I always use as a dressing.

I put in whatever cold vegetables I have and maybe a bit of grated leek or onion and lettuce if I have it. If not, I cut up some cabbage finely and perhaps a carrot. I wonder what you have? Every day we should eat some raw food because it is full of minerals that keep our bones strong. You may have heard of older people having 'brittle bones' and so getting a broken bone if they fall. Raw vegetables help to cure this and I find I enjoy a raw salad in winter as well as in summer.

You can mix some boiled cold rice in with it, or some macaroni. You can get pasta in all sorts of fancy shapes nowadays. Or if you have scraps of fish or chicken, try adding those. Personally, I make my salads in a bowl, not on a plate. It is then easier to mix it all up. If you leave it for some minutes before you eat it, the flavours mix together and it tastes delicious.

We are told that we should have some bulk in our food to prevent constipation and to keep all our digestion really active. So every day we need some potatoes, rice, any kind of beans, wholemeal brown bread, any sort of pasta, barley or nuts.

I make Scotch broth very often in winter. I am Scottish so we always had it at home. A bone from a lamb joint is the correct stock but nowadays I may use a stock cube, some barley that has been steeped overnight and any kind of chopped up vegetable. Add some raw parsley just before eating. It is scrumptious and very filling. Try it with a lump of crusty brown bread, preferably warm and crisp.

The doctors say we should not have too much fat, sugar or salt. So I have skimmed milk, low fat spread and I never buy biscuits or cakes.

You will find, I think, the more sweet things you eat, the more you want. And who wants to get fatter and fatter? I don't, so I only have a piece of cake or chocolates when I am out to tea.

By the way, I hope you often ask friends to share your meals or, if you live in a home with others, I hope you make meals a time for friendly chat and not just sit there munching in silence. You will find you enjoy your meal more if there is a laugh with it. So it may be up to you to start some conversation at your table.

Now drinking! I'll take a bet you don't drink three to four pints every day. But that is the amount you need to balance the thin part of your blood, flush out your kidneys which clean your blood, and also provide for sweating.

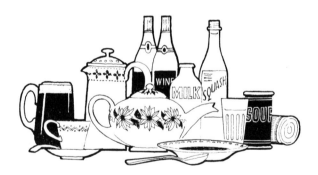

You may think you never sweat, or perspire, often people tell me that, but everybody does. In fact, it is by sweating that the body keeps its temperature level. This is called 'invisible sweat' and that is why we are often not as aware of it as we are when we get very hot and sweat pours down our faces. Some people forget about that invisible sweat and so they don't bother to wash all over every day, or better still, have a bath or shower.

Please do drink enough for the benefit of your whole body. Any healthy fluid will do. Some tea and coffee, a little wine or beer, water, soup, fruit juices. There are so many delicious drinks, we can all find something we like, so there is no excuse for not drinking enough – but not sweet, fizzy stuff please.

Skin is a living thing. It covers the fatty layer which is all over our bodies and the skin itself grows over this in a layer of living cells. As these cells multiply from below, they get pushed up towards the surface, gradually getting more squashed until finally the top layer is actually dead skin.

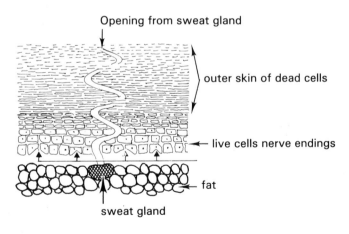

Opening from sweat gland

outer skin of dead cells

live cells nerve endings

fat

sweat gland

I am sure sometimes you have rubbed off some dry skin. Well, every day we should be rubbing all our withered skin away with a good old rub with a towel, after using a well-soaped loofah or rough sponge to freshen up our skin.

Many people like to use a freshener with a smell that they like, or talcum powder afterwards. This is a good idea. If you have a very dry skin you may prefer a sweet-smelling lotion. How pleasant it is to go into a room full of people and find it smelling fresh and pleasant; and how horrid it is to smell that stale smell of unwashed people and old fusty clothes.

▤ Deep breathing and coughing

You may have noticed that I often mention breathing. This is because it is so important to get rid of the gas given off by all the cells of your body as waste, and to supply these same cells with plenty of oxygen which they use as fuel when they are working. This they do all day long, so all day long, your blood has to be pumped by your heart through your lungs, to get rid of the acid gas (carbon dioxide) and to find the supply of oxygen.

This takes place in the tiny air passages in your lungs as the fresh air comes in. These passages are so fine and so numerous, that if you spread them all out they would cover a tennis court. Just think of that, a tennis court!. So it seems a pity not to use such a vast area fully when we have it; your brain in particular demands oxygen to work with. If it is starved of oxygen for four seconds, you can get brain damage, and if it doesn't get oxygen for four minutes, you are dead!

So let us think about it.

Your chest is shaped like this

a rib just like the
handle of a bucket
or pail

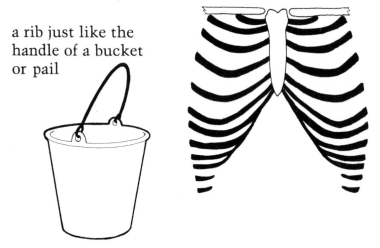

and your ribs can move sideways up and down just
like the handle of a bucket, because they are
attached at the back to your spinal bones, and in
front to your breast bone, and so the middle part
can move freely.

If you never breathe deeply they don't get a chance
to move, and you very easily get short of breath.

Underneath your lungs your diaphragm is shaped
like an umbrella with its handle attached inside
low down to your spinal bones and with its edges
attached all round the lower ribs. The lungs sit on
top of this umbrella with your heart between
them slightly to the left. When the diaphragm
works, the middle part lowers, pressing
downwards and then it heaves out the ribs.

Because the ribs are attached to the lungs on the
inside, the lungs are therefore stretched, and their
passages opened. This makes the outside fresh air

rush into the lungs.

When you breathe out, the diaphragm rises and the ribs fall back against the lungs. This pressure from all sides presses out your stale air.

Good, thorough breathing is slow – about twelve times a minute. Don't hold your breath. If you find you do, just breathe out and you will find you always breathe in again.

■ Good breathing

Put your hands gently around your lower ribs with the tips of your fingers just touching in front.

Gently breathe in through your nose, letting your tummy expand; fingers should be moved slightly forwards. *(1)* Go on breathing in. Your hands will be pushed sideways as your ribs rise outwards and upwards like the bucket handle. *(2)(3)* Go on breathing in at the top of your chest.

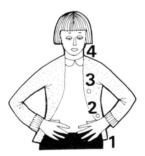

Continue breathing in and try and feel the air right behind your nose. *(4)*

Do all this in your own time and then gently breathe out through your nose, and you will feel your ribs drop downwards and inwards. You can give them a little push with your hands in that direction, if you like. Then breathe in again when you are ready.

You should always breathe in and out through your nose as it is specially arranged inside for this. It is lined with sticky fluid to catch any dirt in the air, and also has warm blood vessels near its surface to warm the air as it passes along, just like central heating pipes. You therefore have cleaned and warmed air before it reaches your lungs.

If you breathe through your mouth none of this happens, and your lungs really prefer the clean, warmed air they get if you breathe through your nose.

If you feel giddy when doing breathing, just let your breath find its own level, stop directing it and forget about it for a while. You have a magnificent area in your brain to look after your breathing, so just leave it in control.

Every day please go outside and take two or three deep breaths. If it is very cold wrap up. Deep breathing in fresh air is a wonderful tonic.

■ Useful coughing

I wonder if you know what a cough is for? It is to bring up any deposit in your breathing tubes, so that you can then spit it out. Do this into a paper tissue, and then dispose of it.

If you do not do this, then you should not be coughing. Some people cough from habit and give themselves a sore throat, some people have an irritable throat and need a soothing syrup ordered by the doctor.

But if you have a deposit that you can hear rattling in the back of your throat, here is how to get rid of it gently and easily. You will then be able to breathe better, and with less distress.

□ Sit down with your back supported, and put your hands as before around your lower chest.

□ Slowly take a deep breath in, as already described.

□ Hold your breath for a moment, then open your mouth wide and cough out in an explosive, noisy gust – only one large explosion should bring up the phlegm, but if it doesn't, just sit and breathe quietly and then try again. You will soon learn the trick of how to do it.

□ Don't struggle. Keep calm.

It usually works, and when I used to teach this cough to patients troubled by sticky phlegm, it was lovely to see the relief on their faces after they had brought it up so easily, and thus got rid of it and their continuous irritating cough.

▤ Make a strong back

□ Press your head back against the chair. Do this three times, *PRESS BACK, STOP, PRESS BACK, STOP, PRESS BACK, STOP.*

□ Now stick your nose up in the air so you look at the ceiling and continue pressing back against the chair, *PRESS BACK, STOP, PRESS BACK, STOP, PRESS BACK, STOP.*

☐   Leave your head on the back of the chair with your nose pointing forward; roll your head from side to side. Now raise one arm, it doesn't matter which, put your hand on the top of your head and press your elbow as hard as you can towards the chair back three times as before.

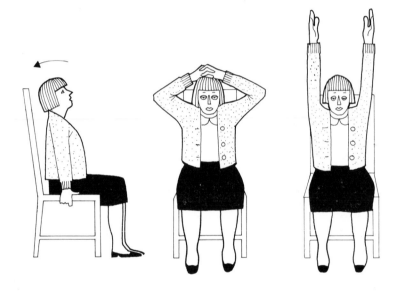

☐   Stretch your hand up to straighten your arm so that your hand points to the ceiling and again do the pressing back with your whole arm. Lower your arm very slowly down till it rests on the arm of your chair.

Have a little rest and then repeat the whole performance with your other arm, and finally with both arms.

☐ Now push your leg forwards – it doesn't matter which – with your heel on the ground and your toes pointing to the ceiling. Really push it out from your body till your knee is quite straight. Lift your leg as though you were giving a little kick with the toe of our shoe.

☐ *GO ON, KICK! KICK! KICK!*

☐ Then drag your heel back again on the floor to where it started with your toes pointing downwards. Repeat it all again with your other leg. Have a rest.

When you feel ready to have another go, sit forwards in the chair so that your bottom is at the front of the chair and your feet are firmly on the ground, a little distance apart.

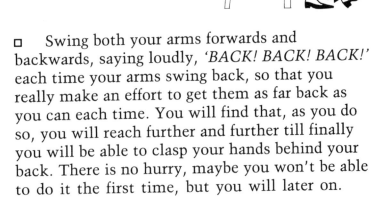

☐ Swing both your arms forwards and backwards, saying loudly, *'BACK! BACK! BACK!'* each time your arms swing back, so that you really make an effort to get them as far back as you can each time. You will find that, as you do so, you will reach further and further till finally you will be able to clasp your hands behind your back. There is no hurry, maybe you won't be able to do it the first time, but you will later on.

When you can clasp your hands together, try

moving them up and down your back. This movement will help you to put your arm into a sleeve of a dress or jacket which maybe, at the moment, you find difficult. Little and often is the answer. Always stop when you feel tired, you can try again later.

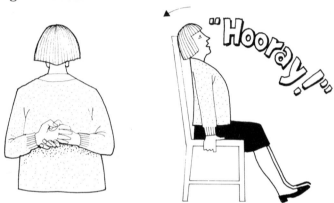

Finally, push both your legs forwards on the floor, clasp your hands on your chair and bend your head backwards as far as you can, all at the same time. Try to see the ceiling. When you can do all this together, call out 'HOORAY!' You deserve it.

▤ Dealing with incontinence

Incontinence has been called 'a very common complaint'. It means the inability to control the flow of urine from the bladder or the contents of the bowel, or sometimes both.

This difficulty affects thousands of people, and has the most serious consequences, both emotional and social.

The first thing to say is that it can always be managed, so that the person concerned can lead a more comfortable life. However, there is so much shyness and shame connected with this difficulty, that often the unfortunate person simply puts up with it – even tries to hide it. Often their family and friends don't realise there is anything wrong, until they notice a fusty smell around the person, and wonder why they never want to go out.

But this is a medical condition, like measles or a cold in the head. It's nothing to be ashamed of, so the secrecy is quite unnecessary. The best thing to do is to tell your doctor of your difficulty. He or she will not be at all surprised, as so many people have this problem.

He or she may refer you to a 'Continence Advisor'. They are now specially trained to help, and are found all over the country, and will sort out what is the best plan for you. You might be sent to a specialist physiotherapist, as often exercise and advice can cure the condition completely, even after years of trouble.

In the meantime you may want to understand the area we are talking about. It is the lowest area inside the pelvis where there are the exits from the bladder and bowel. It is composed of skin, muscle and fat just like any other part of our bodies, and is called 'the pelvic floor'.

The muscles are mostly small, interwoven with each other, and bulging slightly downwards but acting as a sling to support the contents of the pelvis. There is some tightening around the exits.

In both men and women, around the exit from the bowel, there is a tight ring called the anus which should only let go at will to let the contents come out. Further forwards, in women, there is the opening called the vagina, where intercourse takes place, and through which a baby is born, so often it remains stretched afterwards.

Further in front, in both men and women, is the exit from the bladder with of course different shapes, but both controlled by muscle which should be under the control of the will.

If this whole area becomes stretched it will obviously mean that these exits also tend to become stretched and therefore the contents leak out at any time. Extra fat is a cause of stretching, as is also sitting or lying motionless for long periods of time.

Now muscle doesn't like being stretched. Its business is to contract, that is to get smaller, and as so many people don't realise they have a pelvic floor, they therefore don't know how to make it work. Remember it is made of ordinary muscle like that controlling your limbs or your face.

◻ Purse up your mouth like this. Keep it tightly closed and at the same time tighten up your anus at the other end. Go on – tighten up below. Please don't be shy, we are all made exactly the same. Tighten more and more, then rest and I'll explain the next part of the exercise called 'Tightening the pelvic floor' or 'Pelvic floor tensing'.

□ From the anus forwards, you draw up the fat and the skin upwards inside you, and you try to squeeze it altogether upwards.

□ Try now. Lift your inside pelvic floor upwards away from the seat of your chair and then squeeze hard – lift and squeeze, go on squeezing tightly and breathe out strongly as you do so.

You should not squeeze your buttocks together, they are outside muscles and you are learning to contract and strengthen inside muscle. Rest.

Repeat all this as often as you wish, sitting or standing, whenever you remember. You will be delighted to find that you can often cure yourself by doing this pelvic floor tensing exercise.

Try also, when you are passing urine, to stop and start the stream several times. If you can do this, you will gradually tighten the control of the muscles guarding the exit and you will increase their strength so that you do not leak. This is always a tremendous triumph and anyone, man or woman, who achieves it is justly proud of themselves. So keep at it.

But please, do also ask for help. If you are shy of going to your doctor by yourself, tell someone you know well, and ask them to go along with you. There are also a number of good publications on incontinence – see the book list at the back of this book.

Remember everyone at some time has 'wet' themselves, perhaps when coughing or laughing suddenly. Coughing especially can cause leaking.

Your Mind

▤ Think Free

There are some people who spend a lot of time in wheelchairs, others who are in bed and some who do not leave their homes. These people are often spoken of as:

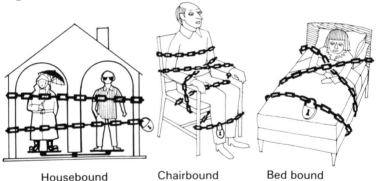

Housebound   Chairbound   Bed bound

Isn't it ridiculous? Of course they aren't chained! Just because they spend a lot of time in a chair or bed or house doesn't mean they are bound to them!

So if you are one of these people, object to these horrid terms. Don't let people use such stupid language about you. Laugh at them! It is only sloppy thinking on their part.

If people are so silly, we have to demonstrate to them by our own attitude and they way we live, that we are not bound to anything. I cannot walk without the help of a crutch, but no one is allowed to call me 'crutchbound'.

Here are a few ideas how you can demonstrate your independence.

☐　The most important thing is to *THINK FREE*. Remember you have a mind and spirit as well as a body, and your mind and spirit can soar to any heights and any distance no matter where your body may be.

☐　Practise independence of thought. Be yourself. Don't just accept other people's opinions and certainly not their orders, unless you agree with them. It is so easy to be dismissed into some little bundle of humanity as though you hardly existed as a person.

☐　Correct people if they use these horrid words about you. There is a programme on the radio called 'Does He Take Sugar?' which is such a clever way of indicating how disabled people are often ignored in their presence, and questions they could answer are addressed to someone else. So don't let it happen to you. Speak up for yourself.

☐　Then you must demonstrate freedom. I heard about a wonderful man breaking the 5000 metres world paraplegic record at the world wheelchair games in 1987. He is certainly not chairbound!

You may not be able to join in races, but there is always some activity you can practise daily to increase what you can do. So work at it. *'USE IT OR LOSE IT'* is the slogan to remember.

☐ Accept responsibility for yourself in every way you can. Washing, dressing, moving about. Sometimes you really have to stop other people taking over. 'It is quicker' they say if they dress you, for instance. Well, you have the time, you do it. Let them leave your clothes beside you for you to dress in your own time and pace. I have found a magic phrase to stop other people taking me over – *'I CAN MANAGE, THANK YOU'*. Try it.

☐ Think about what you can do for others. Surely every adult person should be doing something for someone else? Only animals and children are continually being the receivers of attention.

☐ Would you like a pen friend or perhaps to join your local church or other religious group, or even a political party? Whether or not you actually visit them, you will certainly be welcome as a member, and there are always jobs to be done that you can do at your own pace.

☐ Jumble sales, village fetes and amateur dramatics can be the greatest fun to join in if you can possibly get there. If you can't, then offer to make out lists, address envelopes, paint scenery, sew costumes, bake a cake, make sandwiches, create headdresses or draperies. The possibilities are endless if you are determined to *THINK FREE*.

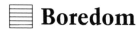 Boredom

Do you ever mutter those dread words 'I'm so bored'? Everybody has at some time or another, and what a waste it is of the limited precious time we have at our disposal.

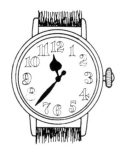

Surely that is the important thing to remember. *TIME IS OURS*. We can plan it however we choose. If we don't use it for interest and enjoyment for ourselves or others, it is our fault – no one else's – no one can take it from us.

Boredom is a killer. Why? Because then everything in your body slows down as you sit around motionless and unthinking. As it slows, it tends to become unhealthy. Indigestion, constipation, wind, chest complaints, headaches, weak legs, clogged arteries, these may be the result of wrong diet, sitting still and getting gradually more and more bored with everything, and everybody.

Of course, it takes an effort sometimes to find something interesting to do, but it is so worthwhile. But this is true for everyone, so don't you be the one who doesn't try! Just begin with attending to your own body (page 75), your own food and drink (page 35) and smarten up your own clothes (page 67).

That will lead you on to other interesting occupations, especially when people compliment you and say how well and how nice you look.

Maybe you could find some compliments to give to a friend, or one of your own family? Do try to say something pleasant to them and just watch them beam with pleasure. 'Spread a little happiness, as you go by!'

So the answer is – *PLAN*, *PLAN*, *PLAN AHEAD*, and choose something you really want to do with your most precious possession, Time.

If you like long telephone talks with your friends or family, that's a splendid way to use your time, but there are some people who use the telephone as a kind of weapon to bully us, and they go on boring us with repetitive, uninteresting chatter.

Learn to get away if you want to, you don't have to stand there listening if you don't enjoy it. Just say 'I'll have to go now, perhaps we'll have a talk another time', and that's it. You can think of other suitable farewells yourself.

There are so many other ways that you find your time taken from you. You may be expected to sit still with other people doing nothing for hours, or watching continuous television that has no interest for you.

Don't agree to it. You can quite politely say you would rather do something else. Go off and do it, even if it is only a walk in the garden or along a corridor. But I hope you have other interesting ploys on hand.

So what do you do with the time you have now at your own disposal? Perhaps you can remember something you used to enjoy doing and have forgotten about. Did you once enjoy knitting, sewing, reading, painting, baking, bottling fruit, dancing, walking? Would it be possible to begin again at your favourite thing? Discuss it with some sympathetic, understanding person. Or you might try a completely new hobby. It is exciting that we have so much choice.

If you find plenty of variety in your life, and enjoy sharing what you are doing with others, you will be an interesting person yourself, and people will like being with you. One thing leads to another. Suppose you learn to make stuffed soft toys, soon you find yourself being asked to join in at some church sale, or Women's Institute, to sell them, or you organise a raffle of your best toy for your favourite charity. Soon you find yourself being invited to some function when you present your cheque to the charity officials, and so on.

There is such a variety of adventures ahead, you could fill your life ten times over.

☰ Stress and the Mitchell Method of Relaxation

I discovered this method of relaxation in 1957 when I had trouble with displaced discs in my arthritic neck. Since then the method has been used all over the world, and is much used in our own National Health Service. I would like to explain it briefly in this book for anyone who is suffering from stress.

Stress is caused by some part of the way a person lives which troubles them, and which they cannot or will not change. Sometimes people are not aware of the actual cause of their stress, and become really ill. Always the best thing to do is to think out the cause and, if at all possible, deal with it. Perhaps by discussing it with a friend.

During stress, the body is in a state of 'fight or flight' dominated by extra activity of certain glands.

Part of the state of tension is the positioning of the whole body in a punching, defensive position. Hands are clenched and may clasp each other or something else; the arms bend up and hug the body; the body and head tend to bend forwards; if sitting, the legs cross, or instead the person may walk about continuously; the breath is often shallow or held and then let out in gusts.

One way to cut through this exhausting state of *'FIGHT OR FLIGHT '* is to change this position to exactly the opposite position, joint by joint. The result is Total Relaxation.

This causes the heart to slow down, the blood pressure to lower and the blood to flow easily to all parts of the body so that they all work normally.

This is a great relief to the person, as I have seen in literally thousands of people during the last thirty years in which I and others have been teaching this method.

We simply follow the rules by which the body changes any position to another position. These rules are the physiology of the body, that is how all parts of the body work. These rules never change and when they are not obeyed the whole person tends to become ill in body, mind or spirit, or to have a general breakdown.

You change the position of tension to relaxation by the following method:

1 You give yourself an order to change position in one area (see below).

2 You **STOP** doing that movement.

3 You feel the resulting position in your joints and in the pressure on your skin.

The result is Relaxation and a lovely sense of comfort. You will probably prevent yourself from getting ill if you practise this every day.

What you must not do are the following:

□ Do not give orders to muscles, eg say 'relax' or try to feel relaxation there. This is because muscles do not have direct contact with your brain. The brain gives orders only for action and the muscle work is learned by doing the action, eg drink you tea, drive the machine, etc.

In the same way you can feel the pressure on your skin as you hold this book, and also realise the position of all your joints if you give them some attention, but you really cannot feel the tension in the actual muscles, so don't try. You have not got the nerves to convey this information.

☐   Do not change the Self orders. I have worked them out because of a law of the body whereby, if you give an order which results in the working of one group of muscles, the group that does the opposite work then automatically lets go, ie relaxes.

So if your hands are grasped tightly like this

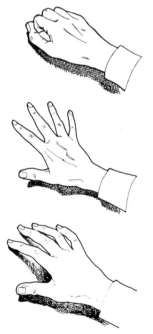

and you give yourself the order *'open out and stretch your fingers'* like this

you get an automatic relaxing of the muscles that clench up your fingers. You then say *'STOP'* and the muscles opening your fingers stop working, and the fingers fall back onto their support like this

So now all the muscles controlling your hands are relaxed and resting. You then spend some time feeling the new position of your joints, and the touching on your skin so that in the future you can recognise a tense hand and you know how to relax it. It is really very simple if you follow the rules. Do it often and you will soon find it quite easy, and I know you will like the result.

Before we begin, get yourself into a suitable position. Either lie down on your back on the floor with a pillow under your head; or sit up in bed supported on pillows; or sit in a chair with a tall back and side arms putting your arms on the chair arms; or you can sit leaning forward onto pillows on a table with your head resting on your arms comfortably placed on the pillows. The orders will fit any position, that is another reason why you must not alter them. They are very exact and in every day language.

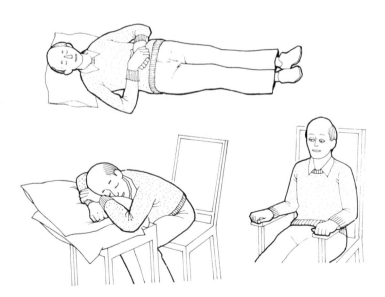

Shoulders

Self order: 'Pull your shoulders towards your feet'. Don't drop them, really pull them strongly away from your ears. *STOP* They will bounce to their own comfortable position.

Feel The tops of your shoulders are further away from your ears.

Elbows

Self order: 'Elbows out and open'. Keep your arms on the support and push your elbows slightly away from your sides. *STOP* Then open out your elbow joints slightly. *STOP*.

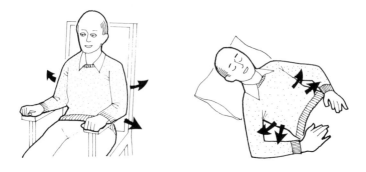

Feel Your arms are touching heavily on the support, floor, bed, table etc with the elbows away from your sides and elbow joints open rather than bent up.

Hands

Self order: 'Stretch your fingers and thumbs out long and open, and bend the hands back at

your wrists'. *STOP* Your hands
will fall onto the support.

Feel Your fingers are
separated, your finger
tips are touching chair,
pillow, sheet, skirt or
trousers on your tummy,
nails are on TOP.

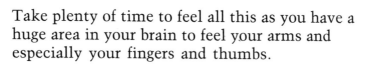

Take plenty of time to feel all this as you have a
huge area in your brain to feel your arms and
especially your fingers and thumbs.

Legs

Self order: 'Turn your legs outwards'. *STOP*
Your knees now face to the sides like
Charlie Chaplin.

Feel The new position.

Knees

Self order: If you are
sitting, if your knees are not
comfortable, move them
gently till they are
comfortable and then *STOP*.

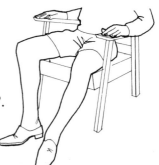

Feel The comfort you have
produced.

Feet

Self order: 'Push your feet away from your face' because tense feet tend to come upwards. *STOP*.

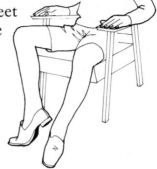

Feel Your feet are dangling.

Body

Self order: 'Push your body into the support'. *STOP*.

Feel Your body is touching the support forwards, backwards or sideways depending how you are lying.

Head

Self order: 'Push your head into the support'. This is always in the same direction as your body. *STOP*.

Feel: Your head is touching the support; its weight is being taken there. Your head weighs nearly as much as a stone of potatoes! So feel it lying supported, and all the muscles in your neck will relax.

Breathing

Self order: 'Gently breathe in through your nose, expanding your tummy and all your ribs, then breathe gently out again through your nose'. Only do this twice. Do not force.

Face

Now we come to the beauty treatment. Remember your self order always tells you to do an exact movement, so you say:

Self order: 'Drag down your jaw'. Do not drop it. Just lower it down enough to separate your teeth, with your mouth closed gently. *STOP.*

Feel Your separated teeth, your easy lips gently touching each other, and put your tongue in the middle of your mouth, with the tip touching the lower teeth. You have now given yourself a relaxed mouth; so concentrate on your lips, your teeth, and your tongue, and you will find your saliva will then flow freely. Now you know what to do if you have a dry mouth.

Eyes

Self order: 'Close your eyes'. You may already have shut your eyes. If so, that is splendid because your brain has by now received so many messages of comfort that it may have closed your eyes to help you relax more. Do not screw up your eyes at all, you only lower the top lids then *STOP.*

Feel The lovely darkness you have made for yourself. Enjoy it.

Forehead

Think of smoothing your forehead up into your

hair, then pushing your hair over the top of your head and down the back of your neck. When you get good at this you will actually feel your hair move. This means the tight muscle under your scalp has let go.

Your mind

Please stay where you are lazily and luxuriously feeling all your joints and noticing their comfortable positions. Then you may go to sleep if you wish, or if you only wish to relax for a short . time, you could repeat all the orders to yourself all round your body. Or if you are quite comfortable, choose some happy memory to occupy your mind, and think about it slowly, remembering every detail you enjoyed.

When you are ready, stretch all over and get up slowly; sit up for some minutes before you stand.

Your Emotions

Clothes and comfort

Let's talk about clothes – day clothes, bed clothes and outside clothes.

■ Day clothes

Do you look over your day clothes, both for inside and outside wear, every spring and autumn? If you do this, you can put aside jumpers, dresses, a jacket perhaps, or slacks that have seen a lot of wear or that you have tired of, or never really liked. Give them away! You can always find a jumble sale that will be delighted to have them. Or you may know someone you can swop with; or go on an expedition with a friend to buy something new. Do choose a colour you really enjoy. Try it up against your face and look in the mirror to see if it suits your skin colour, and your eyes. Never mind fashion. Choose for your own taste and then other people will appreciate the result as part of your personality.

If you find it difficult to go out, try using a mail

order service. There are many of these; ordering is easy, and they all offer to change garments if not suitable, or to refund money. You can get underwear or top clothes and many kinds of gadgets and pretty or useful things suitable for Christmas or birthday presents.

Remember everyone else has to look at you, so it is worth taking great trouble to be as attractive as possible. Some people choose dull colours because, they say, 'It doesn't show the dirt'! What a pity! Much better to wear things that do show the dirt, and then you can tell when they need washing.

It is a great boost to your own confidence to change into some freshly-washed and ironed shirt or blouse, or woollie. With all the new washing powders and materials, this is so much easier. Look at the label and you may find you needn't even iron – just wash, rinse and hang up to dry.

Do try to vary what you wear in spring, summer, autumn and winter. This doesn't mean you have to have a vast wardrobe, it just means you do get a change and a change does us all good. Put the clothes you are not wearing carefully away wrapped up against moths. I haven't much cupboard space but I put these things in a suitcase under my bed. Some have been in and out for thirty years!

In this way you will find you welcome favourite clothes, year after year, because you only use them for a few months at a time – and just listen to the compliments you meet!

■ Winter comfort

Fishermen know all about winter comfort and if you look at them, you will find they wear *LAYERS*. Much better than one thick woollie is to have several layers, both of underwear and top clothes. Wool of course is wonderful but some man-made fibres are just as warm if you choose carefully. Keep your head, hands, feet and legs warm, because your body heat escapes from them very easily. People who can knit, crochet, or sew have a great advantage, so if you have once made woollies or clothes I do hope you have kept it up.

If you have stopped, perhaps because you have poor eyesight or arthritis, why not begin again? You can get quite strong spectacles or even a magnifying glass to hang around your neck.

Try a long shawl or scarf on big pins; then, when you get good at it, you might go on to leg warmers, mittens, bed socks or even a bed hat. Think how pleased you will be to have achieved something really pretty and useful for yourself! So much more amusing than sitting all day with your hands getting stiffer and your mind bored.

Try to go out every day, unless of course it is thick snow, or too slippery to walk safely. Then try to get on a porch or balcony just to get the benefit of the bracing air. Wear all your warmest clothes, even if it is only for five minutes, and if there's an icy

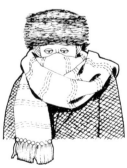

wind, breathe through a woollen scarf across your face.

It is most important in winter to get into a warm bed. Don't let a cold bed steal your body heat. See that the window is closed. Yes *CLOSED*. The old-fashioned Victorians opened their windows three inches at night and made a fine freezing draught; but they had layers of heavy curtains and stuffy furniture.

Nowadays it is wiser to open your windows in the day to air the room, then shut them at night. Don't be like those silly people coughing continuously and saying *'BUT I ALWAYS SLEEP WITH MY WINDOW OPEN'*. Yes, and they always cough!

I feel sorry for their chests, inflamed, sore and dosed with icy air. What they need is a light shawl or scarf over their head, and warm moist air from a lovely steaming mug of cocoa or soup. This is wonderfully soothing as it slips down your throat, instead of the frosty blast of air. Just try it.

Put a warm pad or hot water bottle in the bed an hour before you intend to go into it. If possible, warm the room, too, with a safe stove. If you have to get up in the night, be sure to put on a warm dressing gown and slippers. I hope you have a light in the passage on the way to the bathroom.

Have you long-sleeved nighties or pyjamas? Have you a woollie hat and a shawl to take to bed with you? This can be a great comfort, you can arrange it over your knees, or across your tummy, or tuck it into your back or around your neck. Being cosy is half the battle in having a good night's sleep.

■ Summer comfort

Put away your winter clothes, and get out your summer ones, for both day and night.

In summer get as much fresh air as you can, and wear short sleeves so enough sun can get to your skin to give you the vitamin D that you need, and which it makes for you when it shines on your skin. Of course, you should not bake your skin in hot sun; if necessary smooth some soft cream into the parts that the sun is shining on.

If it gets really hot try sleeping with nothing on, and only covered by a sheet. You will find it very refreshing, and you sleep much better.

Try keeping, beside your bed, a bowl of cold water with some perfume that you like added to it, together with some ice if possible.

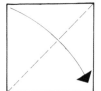 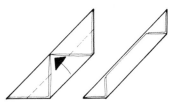

Soak a large handkerchief in it, and then squeeze it out into the bowl and enjoy the fragrance. I put my bowl on a tin tray so that any spilled drops fall onto the tray and not on the furniture. Fold the

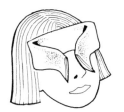

handkerchief on the diagonal twice to make a long bandage. Wave the wet handkerchief in the air to cool it, after your hands have touched it. Spread it across your forehead, and lay the two ends forwards across your eyes, and lie back against your pillows in complete bliss.

You might like to do this for anyone with a headache. They will be very grateful.

▤ The four generations

The four generations of people are: children, young adults, middle-aged adults and elderly people. You and I belong to the last group, but I hope you don't only mix with other older people.

The other groups are so vital to our enjoyment of life as they bring fresh ideas, and quick minds to enliven us. Children I find enchanting. As I have not had any children of my own, not having married, I have to rely on friends' children. I am intrigued by their enthusiasms, and their open ways of talking. They so much enjoy sharing what they enjoy and so do I, so we get along well.

Do you have young visitors? Perhaps you could arrange it, if at the moment you don't. Give it some thought.

When I was ill for some time and could not get out, I gave a set of my front door keys to two families who lived near. They then popped in and out as it suited them, and it made such a lovely surprise when a child brought me the picture she had drawn that day at school, or his page of sums. I am sure their bright chatter helped me to recover as much as the medicines I had to take.

One day I woke from sleep and there beside my bed stood a small pink fairy complete with wings, head dress and wand. As I gazed at her, the fairy's mother came in from the hall and explained that her daughter had been to a fancy dress party, and insisted in coming in to show me her 'sticky-out' dress! Such treats are much more valuable than pep pills.

Everyone has some niggling worry at the back of their mind. It may be quite small like wondering how we can get our shoes mended, to a real scare like wondering how we can pay the next rent due, or some other debt.

The best thing to do is to talk about it to a friend. Someone younger will have enough experience of life to be able to listen with intelligence. It is the *LISTENING* that matters, the best kind of person is not the kind who 'knows all the answers' but one who will listen to you with attention because, in the end, we all have to find our own solutions to our problems; but it is vital to put them into words and gradually, in discussion, we clarify our own minds and can decide our best way out.

Please do not let a false sense of pride stop you from doing this. Everyone has problems, everyone needs friendly talk; perhaps one day you will be able to lend a listening ear to someone else. The more we all share our human dilemmas the better.

The worst thing to do is to bottle up your worries, and go over and over them in your own mind, with your heart sinking as you see no way out.

There is always a way through any difficulty. In fact, whatever is your worry, it has undoubtedly happened many times before. Beware of isolation, that only leads to self-pity and that is so destructive. The answer is always to share, to let a little light in, maybe even to find the humour of the situation.

If you can do all this you will not become like some older people who seem to have developed a grudge against the whole human race and are always bemoaning their ill-luck or ill-health or finding faults in other people.

We all have faults. Let's forget them and nourish the good bits in those around us. There is always plenty to praise if we look for it. A good time really can be had by all.

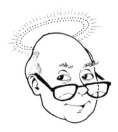

Massage of hands, face and neck

Would you like to have beautiful hands? And face? And neck? Well, you don't have to call in the beauty specialists, or the plastic surgeons, you have the answer in your own hands, and a bottle of scented oil – you choose the scent – or a pot of scented cream.

■ Hands

□ Wash your hands carefully with plenty of soapy lather and scrub your already well-filed nails. Dry them thoroughly.

□ Now sit down with a cushion covered with a fine towel on your knees. Either pour a little oil into one palm, or scoop out some cream from the pot.

□ Now gently rub your palms together, and then spread the oil or cream carefully all over your hands.

□ Rest one forearm on the pillow.

□ Place the thumb and forefinger of the other hand on either side of its thumb. With small circular movements of your finger and thumb gradually press and release your hold on the side of the thumb as you slowly move up the thumb towards your hands.

□   Repeat this along the sides of each finger towards its knuckle which you circle with your thumb. Then knead as before with your finger tips on the back of your hand, while your thumb circles on your palm.

□   Gradually continue in the same way up your forearm to your elbows. You may wish to knead on a return journey to your wrist or else just stroke down and repeat as you wish. Be gentle, slow, careful, and feel a luxurious satisfaction as you work. Finally, change arms on the cushion and massage with the other hand. You may need to add more oil or cream from time to time, if so warm it in your palms before continuing the massage.

■   Face

□   Prepare your hands as before. You should be sitting in a comfortable chair with your head supported backwards on a pillow under your neck.

□   Place the finger tips of both hands pointing upwards on your chin and gradually, making little circular pressing movements, move along your jaws towards your ears.

□   Lift your fingers and place them again on your chin just a little higher up, and repeat as before toward the upper part of your ears.

□   Place your finger tips facing each other in the middle of your forehead and making little circular movements, work towards your hair line at either side. You may have to do this two or three times. It depends on the height of your forehead.

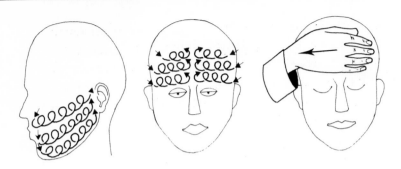

☐   Finally, stroke right across your whole forehead with alternate hands.

☐   Cup both your hands over your two eyes. The hollow of your palms should cover your eyes with your fingers pointing upwards and the heel of your hands resting lightly on your cheek bones. This is a most enchanting feeling, so stay as long as you wish in this position and switch your thoughts to some place or person that gives you pleasure. You might prefer to say a prayer you know and love, or to hum a tune you are fond of. Whatever you do think positively, happily and thankfully.

■ Neck

It is often better to massage the neck at a different time from the hands and face. This is because massage of the neck is rather stimulating, whereas the other is soothing and relaxing. All massage is refreshing because it hastens the blood supply and therefore the supply of oxygen; also because your skin has so many fine nerve endings registering touch and pressure, and these give you emotional satisfaction when gently handled.

▢ Sit in a chair, with a high back, or sit up in bed supported by pillows, with your head resting against one. Press your head backwards once or twice to make sure your head is really leaning on the pillow and then you know that your muscles are relaxed. Never attempt to massage taut muscles, they are still and hard when working and for massage they must feel soft and pliable under your fingers. This is why your head must always be properly supported before you begin to massage your neck.

▢ Oil your hands as before and be sure they are warm. Now lift one hand and place it on the middle of your neck with the fingers pointing towards the opposite ear.

▢ Stroke across quite vigorously away from that ear several times, each time beginning at the middle. Then working in the same direction, knead with your finger tips. Repeat all this with your other hand on the opposite side of your neck. Rest.

▢ When you are ready to begin again, raise both hands, and slip your fingers under your neck, while your head remains resting on its pillow. Place the finger tips low down at the back of your skull. Press as deeply as you can comfortably and knead both sides at the same time, gradually working towards both ears. Return both hands to mid-line, slightly lower and repeat. You can do this several times, gradually working downwards, so that you cover the whole of the back of your neck.

☐   This area is a dense thickened mass of muscles. These are often tired with holding your heavy head up. Did you realise your head weighs about twelve pounds? – that is nearly a stone of potatoes! So it is no wonder your neck needs massage. If your arms get tired, drop one onto your knees and use one had only, then change over. It is quite hard work but your neck will feel so much more comfortable afterwards.

☐   Take a few deep, easy breaths, close your eyes and very gently roll your head from side to side, still supported on its pillow.

☐   You may now want to have a little sleep because you will feel so relaxed and comfortable. Enjoy it.

▦ Care of your feet

It is very difficult to know where to place this section in the book. The obvious place is in the section 'Your Lower Half', but feet are so sensitive, so delicate and so often neglected, that I have decided to put them in the section on 'Your Emotions'.

Feet that receive proper attention and are pampered, as they deserve to be, give great comfort to their owners. Just think of all the work they do for us. That is why they can easily be damaged and cause much discomfort.

■ Shoes

Let us begin with your shoes. Please examine the ones you are using. Are they still a good shape? Long enough? Broad enough? Or have they stretched? What about the linings? Do they need renewing? For winter, you can buy warm slip-in soles and for summer, very thin ones which let the air in. Next examine the heels and underneath the toes. So they need repairing? Many people continue to wear shoes with heels quite worn down at one side. This distorts your walking so much that, not only does it put a strain on your leg muscles and make them ache, but it can even strain your back.

Backache, as a result of ill-fitting shoes, is unfortunately quite common, but many people suffering from it often do not realise the cause.

It may be you should throw out some shoes if they are past repair. Money is well spent on good shoes. Take great care and spend time on fitting and choosing exactly what you want.

Lastly, please polish your shoes with a good polish where possible; brush with a wire brush any suede parts, and renew laces. Smart shoes have a great effect on our sense of well-being.

Your soft slippers should just be for bedroom wear. When you get dressed, always wear proper shoes whether you are going out or not. Your feet will feel much happier in well-fitting proper shoes and you will walk better putting your feet down *HEEL TOE, HEEL TOE*, as you go about the house. People are so apt to shuffle along instead of really lifting their knee on each step and bending the ankle and the foot.

Try also to walk quickly sometimes, walking from room to room or along a passage. It will hurry your heart, your circulation and your breathing, as well as strengthening your feet and legs. Of course be careful not to fall, and be sure there are no loose mats or trailing wires about. Slow walking is often just a bad habit.

■ Stockings, tights, socks and skin

Stockings, socks and tights must be the right length for your feet. If they have shrunk at all, throw them out. They will distort your feet. They should be washed each time they are used because all feet give off quite a lot of sweat. This hardens the soles of your socks and stockings which in turn rubs on the skin of your feet and hardens that. Next thing you know, you have painful hard skin and then corns.

Every day your feet will appreciate being well rubbed with some soothing cream or oil. They should be washed every day as should all your body. So do not soak your feet, this makes the skin too soft. Dry them very thoroughly, especially between the toes.

If possible file your nails and then use an emery board on them. If you can't reach your toes ask someone else to do this for you; but if you do have a corn then you must see a chiropodist. It is dangerous for anyone else to try and cut them and corn pads can also sometimes do harm.

Use animal wool around your toes if they hurt.
You get it from a chemist, tease out a few strands
and wind it around but not too tightly or it will
interfere with circulation. Be sure you wash it
each time you use it. Never use cotton wool, it
forms into little hard balls.

■ **Strengthen your feet**

Sit comfortably, preferably in an upright chair,
with your are feet displayed on a warm rug. Begin
by scrabbling your toes forward so you draw your
foot along the rug. Spread out your toes as widely
as possible and then gently pull your feet back to
where it started with your toes spread out. Toes,
like fingers, are always tending to crumple up.
This way of opening them out strengthens the
supporting muscles and is much safer than pulling
your toes about with your fingers which some
people try to do.

Then, hump up the whole of the middle of your
foot, keeping your toes flat on the ground. Do all
these movements several times as you feel like it,

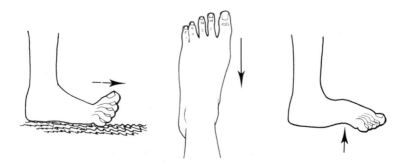

and then bring your foot across your knee, and with well-oiled hands, give it a luxurious careful massage along the sole and top and each toe in turn.

Your feet will thank you, if you really take care of them, by making you feel happier. Let them take you out for a walk every day. Walking is one of the best things you can do for your general health. See that you are wearing suitable clothing for the weather, carry nothing except a stick, or even two sticks if you need them.

Then stride out as freely as possible, swinging your arms if you can. Hold your head high and when you feel like it, take an extra deep breath.

Be sure you have some point in your walk, visit a favourite tree, buy a newspaper or anything else that interests you, but try not to stand about chatting, which is rather tiring. Instead ask you friends to join you in your exhilarating walk.

Your Spirit

▤ The great outdoors

I am writing this leaning the slab of paper on the back of a sleeping cat on my knee. When I wrote other books, I often wrote on a sort of cat sandwich – one on my knee to write on, and one below my chair curled up to keep me company.

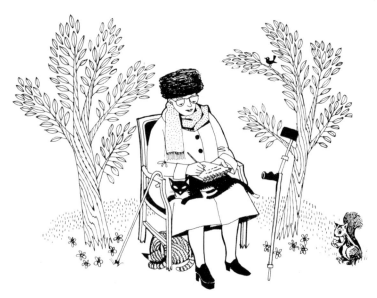

Today it is autumn and I am in the shared garden of the house where I live. Bright yellow and bronze leaves are falling all around. Over there I can see small boys looking for conkers. The sky is blue with white clouds, squirrels are rushing up and down trees with acorns in their mouths. It is cold and I am wrapped up in woollies. Friends pass and call a greeting.

How happy and thankful I am! As I write, I wonder how many people who will read this book, when it is published some time in the future, will also have these pleasures?

PLEASE, PLEASE do take the trouble to use all the chances you have, and all the chances you can make, to enjoy the wonderful world we live in.

Often I have seen people who never left their own home for various excuses, and so their horizons get smaller and smaller, and their interests shrivel accordingly.

'The world is full of a number of things
I'm sure we should all be as happy as kings.'

So let us examine the number of things.

Let's begin with the simplest of all – stones, plants, fish, birds, animals; we share the world we live in with all of these, and surely all of them have much to give us in interest and pleasure, if we will only allow them to do so.

Of course we gain much more if we can go into the world and actively share it by handling and helping in some instances, like caring for plants and trees or appreciating stones by making a wall or a rockery, or even just an edging for a flower bed.

But if we really can't get out we can bring the outdoors indoors. Some people grow cress and make sandwiches for tea, some people grow plants, flowers, even small trees for pleasure; window boxes are getting very popular. Then fish in a tank can give great entertainment and much can be learned about what plants and other creatures get on together.

Many people enjoy keeping a bird; canaries sing, budgerigars have such a variety of colours that I know people find great interest in breeding them.

I have known some people who make a garden in a bottle, and others who create a garden on a tray – moss makes a lawn and a mirror shines as a lake with sand covering all round its edge; living twigs mounted on plasticine are trees and plants.

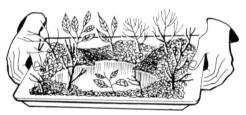

Collecting the materials and arranging and often rearranging them make a fascinating hobby.

Then the animals. As you have realised I am a cat person, but there are dog people, and those who prefer other animals. Doctors tell us that when we stroke an animal our blood pressure tends to become nearer our normal and also that stress is often soothed away. This is especially true of people who live alone, but it has been found helpful also for families and for those who live in homes along with other older people or even in hospital.

Have you heard of the PAT Dog Association? It consists of people who have suitable quiet, friendly dogs and who are willing to take them to call on other people who haven't got a dog and would like to see one.

The dogs walk about on their leads and people pat them and even chat to them. Often it is a great help to someone who is shy or unhappy.

Of course if you are thinking about getting a cat or a dog for yourself, you have to think about it very carefully. Size of animal, cost, expense of food, need for exercise, vet's bills all have to be considered. But if you decide wisely and find the right animal for you, I am sure you will find your life greatly enriched.

I find cats a constant joy. They are so intelligent and devoted, although they are never servile. I love their dignity, their cleanliness and their good manners. They also exercise themselves and enjoy being brushed and groomed. I had a wonderful Siamese cat who lived until he was fifteen. He used to let me cut his nails when they needed it although he grumbled all the time under his breath. He was a dear companion – liked going out for a daily walk with me even in a snowstorm.

Then he would flatten his ears against it and keep close by me. If I sat down he was up on my knee in a flash and buttoned inside my coat till we started walking again. Of course he talked all the time in all his various voices.

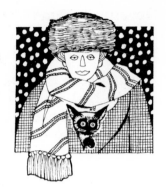

If you are thinking of getting a cat for company, try the Cat Protection League. They have branches all over the country. Volunteers look after stray or unwanted cats and find homes for them with great care. They neuter all cats and kittens who come their way, and see to their general health. I can recommend them.

I do understand what a difficult thing it can be to keep going, and how tempting just to sit still and gaze into space. But I also know that life is so very interesting and amusing; meeting and entertaining people is such a joy that any effort is worthwhile to continue to be part of it and of God's fascinating varied world.

▤ Remembering and appreciating

We older people have very long memories of good patches, and of difficult times, like the wars we have lived through and helped to win. When I watch the Armistice service on the television each

November, I am reminded of the wonderful people I met during the last war, when I worked as a physiotherapist with the wounded.

It is noticeable that each year there are more people, both attending the parade and watching it. Surely this is because we appreciate more and more the preservation of our free way of life which was bought for us by those who died.

It is certainly not a glorification of war, because we remember the horrors of it as well as the joys and friendships. Even the songs the bands play, 'The White Cliffs of Dover', 'Run Rabbit Run', 'We're Going To Hang out the Washing on the Siegfried Line', all bring a lump to our throats, as well as a smile to our lips.

This appreciation of our past experiences is very important to our self-esteem, as well as being our salute to our own generation. While we don't want to dwell unduly on the past, or bore people who cannot possibly understand, it is good to have our private recollections of honouring people we remember.

Then we must find equal interests in the present and appreciate simple, important things like the first snowdrops, a good cup of tea, a warm bath, etc; and we must retain our enthusiasm for making new friends with all that they can give.

Sometimes we are prejudiced against some new experience due to an unhappy time in the past. It is well to examine this quietly by ourselves, or discuss it with someone we can trust. We may well then find that, with hindsight, we can understand the reasons for our unhappiness and forgive those who, probably unconsciously, caused it. This forgiving and forgetting is very valuable to our spiritual well-being. If anyone drags a grudge against the past along with them, they only burden themselves, and may poison their future relationships.

It is sometimes said of older people that they have vivid memories of past events but cannot remember immediate happenings. Often this is true if their present life is both boring and without expectations of any future change or excitement. I have found that, by carrying out some of the previous suggestions, and then consciously creating interest in present day-to-day events, that memory improves considerably.

I'll bet you didn't forget to go to your own wedding! Why? Because you had prepared for it in detail; had looked forward to it, and you knew you looked your best.

If you do all that now in preparing to have a friend to tea, or going out to some event, then you will certainly remember and you will really enjoy it. Interest is the answer.

Of course, everyone forgets things from time to time, especially the young! So don't let anyone say 'What can you expect at your age?' It isn't a problem of old age. It is a question of enjoying life.

Suggestions for further reading

Many of these titles can be bought or ordered from good bookshops or you may be able to borrow them from your local public library. There is often a visiting arrangement or mobile book lending service for older people who can't manage to get to their local branch library. Age Concern England publications can be ordered direct.

Easy Cooking for One or Two by Louise Davies published by Penguin   £2.95

More Easy Cooking for One or Two by the same author, Penguin   £2.95

One is Fun by Delia Smith published by Hodder & Stoughton   £4.95

Eating Well on a Budget by Michael Quinn contains a delicious week's menu for two specially devised by the BBC Food and Drink Programme published by Age Concern England   £1.50

Notes on Incontinence by Dorothy Mandelstam, available from The Disabled Living Foundation, 380/384 Harrow Road, London W9 2HU   £1.20 *including postage.*

Management for Continence by Bob Browne published by Age Concern England   £1.50

What Help is Available? is one of a series of ten free leaflets available from Age Concern England.

Incontinence – a very common complaint is a leaflet from the Health Education Authority obtainable free from local Health Education Units.

Other books by Laura Mitchell

Healthy Living Over 55 published by John Murray in
conjunction with Central Independent
Television *£4.95*

Large print version by ISIS, is now out of print, but can
be obtained from some public libraries.

Simple Relaxation, revised edition 1987, published by
John Murray *£4.95*

Video: 'Life Style, Stress and the Mitchell Method of
Relaxation' by Laura Mitchell, produced by
International Stress and Tension Control Society,
The Priory Hospital, Priory Lane, London SW15 5JJ,
price £19.95.

Other books in this health care series from Age Concern England

The Foot Care Book by Judith Kemp SRCh *£2.95*
A self help guide with advice on routine foot care;
what to do when there is a problem and where to go
for advice. Also included are guidelines about
adaptations and choosing shoes for comfort.

Other publications from Age Concern England

Owning Your Home in Retirement *£1.50*
How to make your home more comfortable and
easy to manage in retirement. Advice on
maintenance, alterations and extensions,
labour-saving fixtures, adaptations and home
security.

Sharing Your Home by Christine Orton £1.95

Many people share their homes happily, but moving in with family or friends, or inviting someone to stay with you, requires serious thought beforehand. This book includes a checklist of financial and legal factors to be considered first, as well as the effect of sharing on state benefits.

A Buyer's Guide to Sheltered Housing £1.50

Buying a flat or bungalow in a sheltered scheme is an option being considered by an increasing number of people, but particular care needs to be taken because of the complicated leasing and management agreements involved. This book covers in detail the points to consider.

Know your Medicines by Pat Blair £3.95

A guide to the medicines commonly used by older people.

At Home in a Home by Pat Young £3.95

Many questions need to be asked when thinking about moving into a residential home. What are the alternatives? What are the pros and cons? What things should I look out for when choosing a home? This practical guide aims to help you make the right decisions regarding a major upheaval in your life.

Age Concern England publications can be ordered direct from The Marketing Department, Age Concern England, 60 Pitcairn Road, Mitcham, Surrey CR4 3LL. Cheques or postal orders should be made payable to Age Concern England and prices include postage and packing.

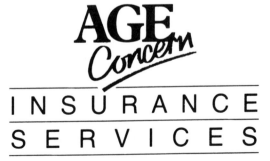

About Age Concern

Age Concern England, the publishers of this book as well as a wide range of others, provides training, information and research for use by retired people and those who work with them. It is a registered charity dependent on public support for the continuation of its work.

The three other national Age Concern Organisations – Scotland, Wales and Northern Ireland together with Age Concern England – form a network of over 1,400 independent local UK groups serving the needs of elderly people, assisted by well over 125,000 volunteers. The wide range of support provided includes advice and information, day care, visiting services, voluntary transport schemes, clubs and specialist facilities for physically and mentally frail elderly people.

Age Concern England
Bernard Sunley House
60 Pitcairn Road
Mitcham
Surrey CR4 3LL
Tel: 01-640 5431

Age Concern Scotland
33 Castle Street
Edinburgh EH2 3DN
Tel: 031-225 5000

Age Concern Wales
4th Floor
1 Cathedral Road
Cardiff CF1 9SD
Tel: 02222 371566/371821

**Age Concern
Northern Ireland**
6 Lower Crescent
Belfast BT7 1NR
Tel: 0232 245729